Paleo Anti-Aging Cookbook

Stay Younger and Energized with these Delicious Recipes

Disclaimer and Terms of Use:

Table of Contents

Introduction

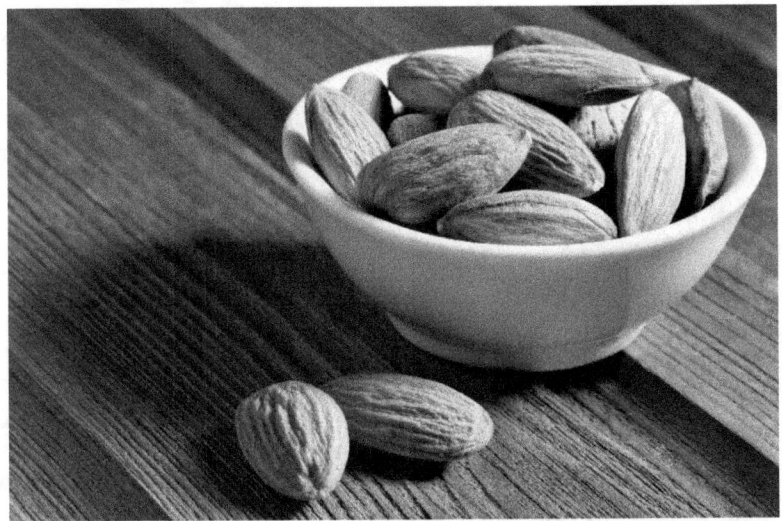

Aging is a fact of life – it happens to everyone and there is nothing you can do to stop it. Just because you can't keep your body from aging, however, doesn't mean that you have to accept the consequences. As you age, your skin starts to wrinkle and sag, your memory starts to slow down, and your joints become stiff. What can you do about it? In addition to taking vitamin and mineral supplements to slow the process of aging, you can also make certain changes to your diet to fight the consequences of getting older.

If you are serious about looking and feeling younger, no matter how old you are, you should consider switching to the Paleo diet. The best thing you can do for your body is to make healthy eating decisions and that is exactly what the Paleo diet is. The Paleo diet is based on the principle of whole food nutrition – it excludes unhealthy processed foods, refined sugars, high-fat dairy products, and packaged convenience foods. In short, the Paleo diet focuses on all of the foods that are good for your body and that will help you to slow down the aging process.

Some of the foods that are best for anti-aging include leafy greens, healthy oils, antioxidant-rich fruits and vegetables, raw nuts and seeds, and lean proteins. All of these foods are included in the Paleo diet. In order to maximize your anti-aging benefits in following the Paleo diet you should exclude dairy products, grains, legumes, and refined sugars and carbohydrates from your diet. When you make positive changes to your eating habits by switching to the Paleo diet you can transform your body and your health, increasing your energy stores and fighting the signs of aging. So, if you are ready to look and feel younger, pick a recipe from this book and give it a try!

Paleo Anti-Aging Recipes

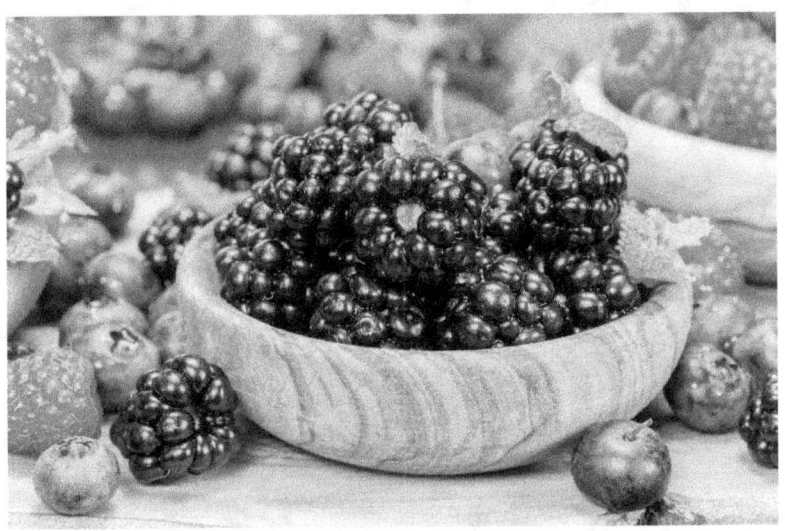

Recipes Included in this Book:

Cream of Broccoli Soup

Strawberry Spinach Salad
with Dressing

Honey Glazed Carrots

Bacon Roasted Brussels
Sprouts

Garlic Mashed
Cauliflower

Roasted Rosemary
Chicken and Veggies

Coconut-Crusted Baked
Halibut

Slow Cooker Beef and
Veggie Stew

Fresh Shrimp Ceviche

Garlic Herb Pork
Tenderloin

Coco-Walnut Baked
Apples

Raspberry Fruit Dip

Dairy-Free Banana Ice
Cream

Blueberry Almond Crisp

No-Bake Coconut Date
Balls

Mushroom and Onion Omelet

Servings: 1

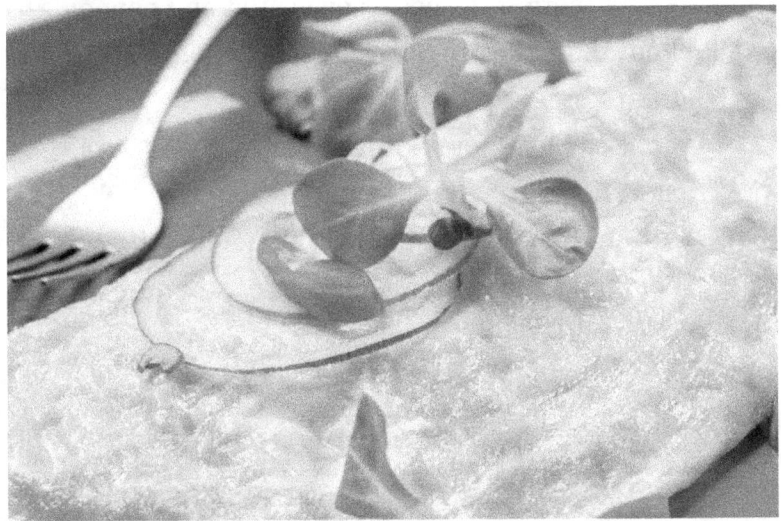

Ingredients:

- 2 teaspoons coconut oil, divided
- ½ cup diced mushrooms
- ¼ cup diced yellow onion
- 1 clove minced garlic
- 2 large eggs
- 1 tablespoon fresh chopped chives
- Salt and pepper to taste

Instructions:

1. Heat 1 teaspoon oil in a small skillet over medium heat.
2. Add the mushroom, onion, and garlic then cook for 3 minutes.

3. Spoon the mushroom mixture into a bowl and reheat the skillet with the rest of the oil.
4. Beat together the eggs, chives, salt and pepper.
5. Pour the eggs into the skillet and cook for 1 minute then stir gently.
6. Cook the eggs for another 2 to 3 minutes until almost set.
7. Spoon the mushroom mixture over half the omelet.
8. Fold the omelet over and cook for 1 minute or until the eggs are set.

Strawberry Banana Breakfast Smoothie

Servings: 1

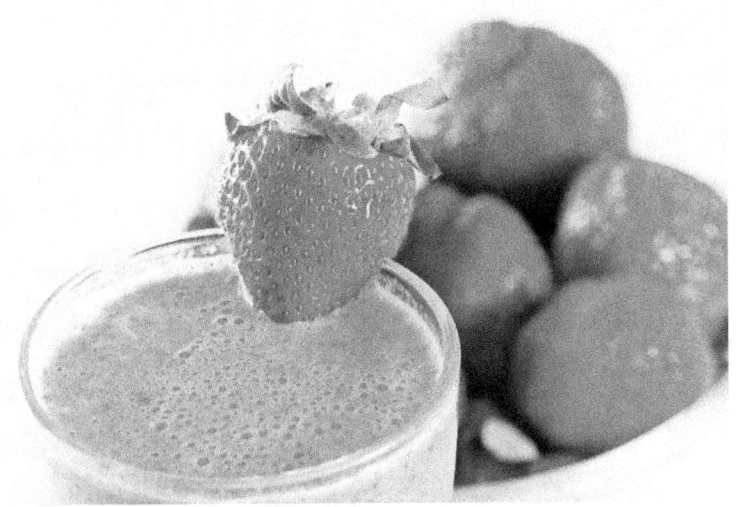

Ingredients:

- 1 cup frozen sliced strawberries
- 1 small frozen banana, peeled and sliced
- 1 handful fresh chopped kale
- 1 cup unsweetened almond milk
- ½ cup ice cubes
- 2 tablespoons almond butter
- 1 teaspoon honey

Instructions:

1. Combine all of the ingredients in a high-speed blender.
2. Blend on high speed for 45 to 60 seconds until smooth and well combined.

3. Pour the smoothie into a glass and serve immediately.

Coconut Banana Pancakes

Servings: 4 to 6

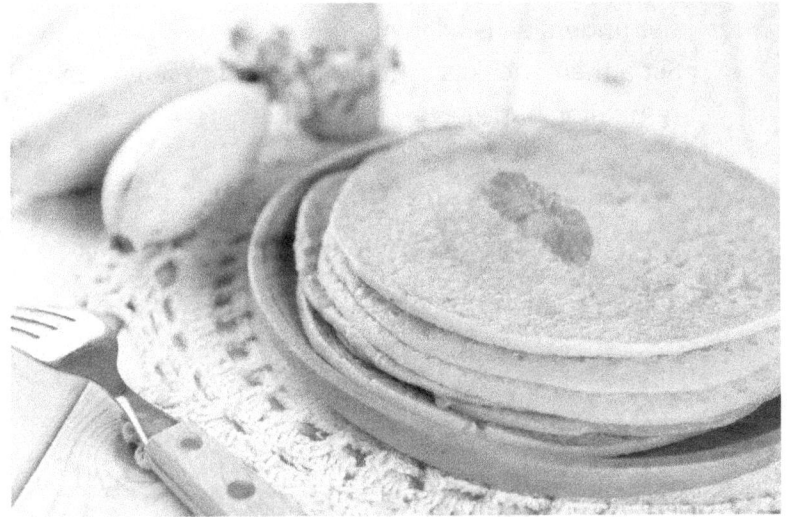

Ingredients:

- 3 large ripe bananas, peeled and sliced
- 6 large eggs, beaten well
- 6 tablespoons sifted coconut flour
- ½ teaspoon ground cinnamon
- Pinch salt

Instructions:

1. Preheat a nonstick skillet over medium heat.
2. Combine the ingredients in a high-speed blender.
3. Blend on high speed for 30 to 60 seconds until smooth.
4. Spoon the batter into the skillet, using about 2 tablespoons per pancake.

5. Spread the batter in a circle then cook until bubbles form in the surface.
6. Flip the pancakes and cook for 2 to 3 minutes until the underside is browned.
7. Slide the pancakes onto a plate and repeat with the remaining batter.

Spinach and Herb Omelet

Servings: 1

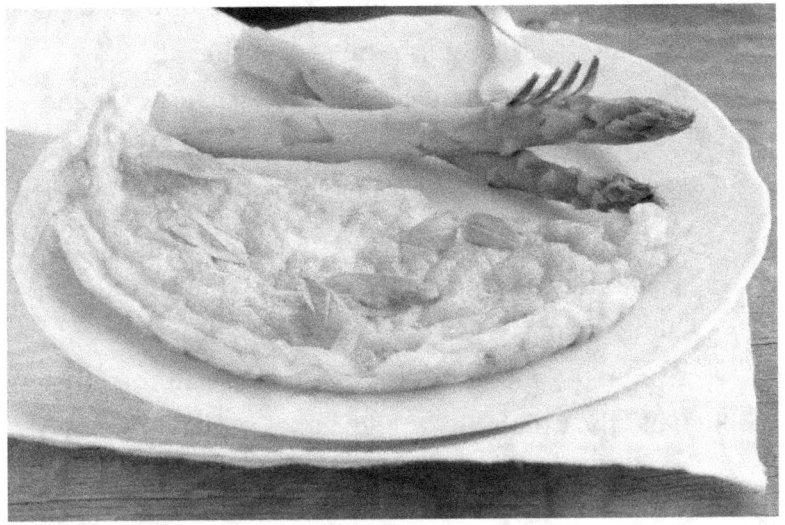

Ingredients:

- 2 teaspoons coconut oil, divided
- 1 cup fresh chopped spinach
- 2 tablespoons diced yellow onion
- 1 clove minced garlic
- 2 large eggs
- 1 tablespoon fresh chopped chives
- 1 teaspoon fresh chopped basil
- ¼ teaspoon dried oregano
- Salt and pepper to taste

Instructions:

1. Heat 1 teaspoon oil in a small skillet over medium heat.

2. Add the spinach, onion, and garlic then cook for 2 minutes.
3. Spoon the mushroom mixture into a bowl and reheat the skillet with the rest of the oil.
4. Beat together the eggs, chives, basil and oregano – season with salt and pepper.
5. Pour the eggs into the skillet and cook for 1 minute then stir gently.
6. Cook the eggs for another 2 to 3 minutes until almost set.
7. Spoon the mushroom mixture over half the omelet.
8. Fold the omelet over and cook for 1 minute or until the eggs are set.

Triple Berry Breakfast Smoothie

Servings: 1

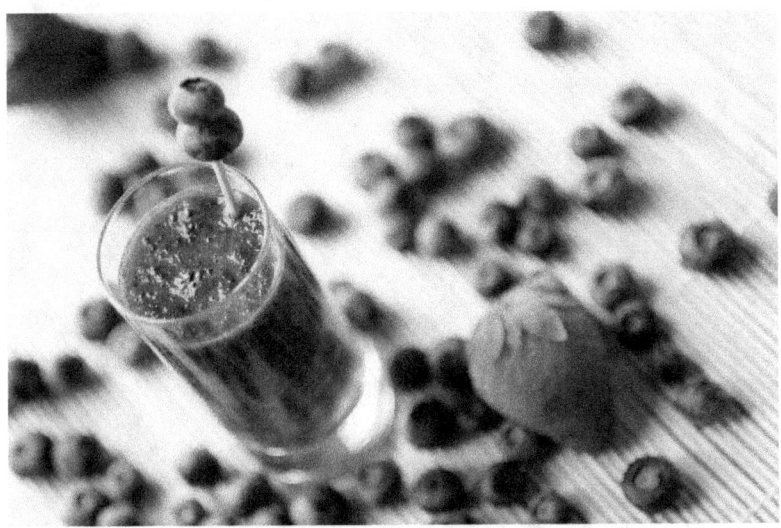

Ingredients:

- 1 cup frozen sliced strawberries
- ½ cup frozen blueberries
- ½ cup frozen raspberries
- 1 cup unsweetened almond milk
- ½ cup ice cubes
- 2 tablespoons ground flaxseed
- 1 teaspoon honey

Instructions:

1. Combine all of the ingredients in a high-speed blender.
2. Blend on high speed for 45 to 60 seconds until smooth and well combined.

3. Pour the smoothie into a glass and serve immediately.

Almond Flour Blueberry Muffins

Servings: 12

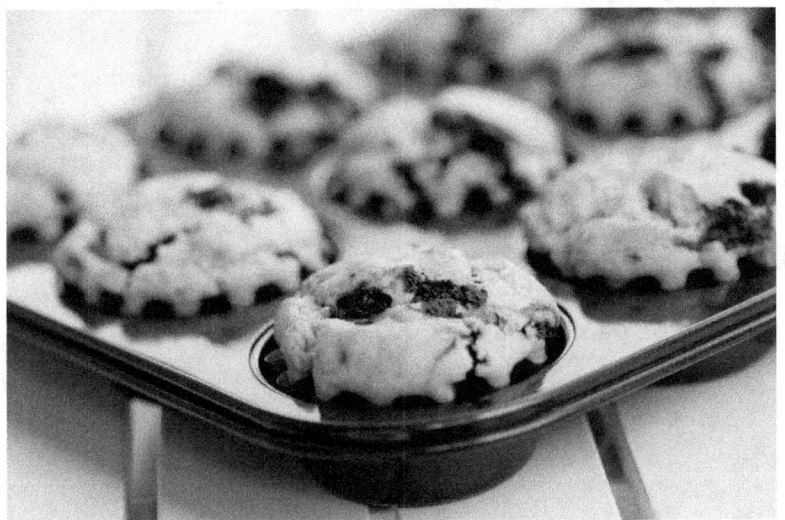

Ingredients:

- 2 ½ cups blanched almond flour
- 1 teaspoon baking soda
- ½ teaspoon ground cinnamon
- Pinch salt
- 1/3 cup unsweetened applesauce
- 2 ½ tablespoons raw honey
- 2 tablespoons melted coconut oil
- 1 teaspoon apple cider vinegar
- 1 teaspoon vanilla extract
- 3 large eggs, beaten well
- 1 cup fresh blueberries

Instructions:

1. Preheat the oven to 350°F and line a muffin pan with paper liners.
2. Combine the almond flour, baking soda, cinnamon and salt in a mixing bowl.
3. In another bowl, whisk together the applesauce, honey, coconut oil, and vinegar.
4. Beat in the eggs and vanilla extract until smooth.
5. Stir the wet ingredients into the dry until well combined.
6. Fold in the blueberries then spoon the batter into the pan, filling the cups ¾ full.
7. Bake for 15 to 18 minutes until a knife inserted in the center comes out clean.

Curried Ginger Soup

Servings: 6 to 8

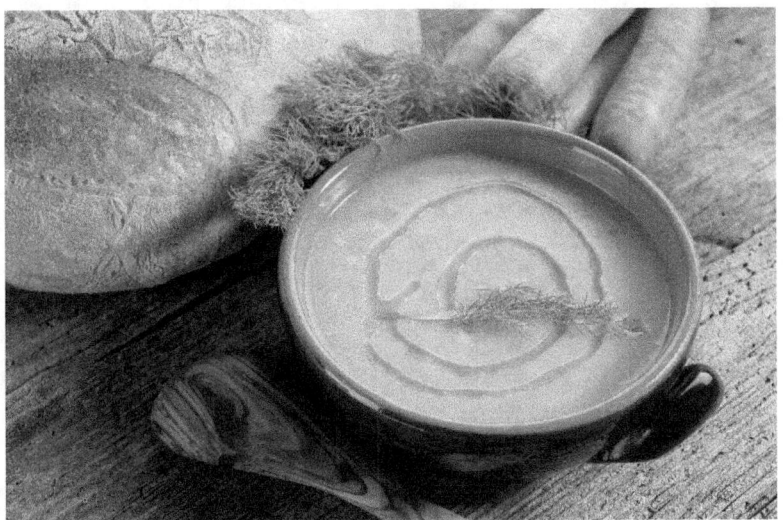

Ingredients:

- 1 tablespoon coconut oil
- 1 small yellow onion, chopped
- 2 lbs. carrots, peeled and sliced
- 1 medium sweet potato, peeled and chopped
- 1 tablespoon fresh grated ginger
- 2 teaspoons curry powder
- 8 cups chicken broth
- Salt and pepper to taste

Instructions:

1. Heat the oil in a large saucepan over medium-high heat.
2. Add the onion and cook for 5 minutes until translucent.

3. Stir in the carrots, sweet potato, ginger and curry powder.
4. Cook for 5 minutes then stir in the chicken broth and bring to a boil.
5. Reduce heat and simmer for 25 to 30 minutes until the carrots are tender.
6. Remove from heat and puree the soup using an immersion blender.
7. Season the soup with salt and pepper to taste – serve hot.

Mediterranean Tuna Salad

Servings: 6 to 8

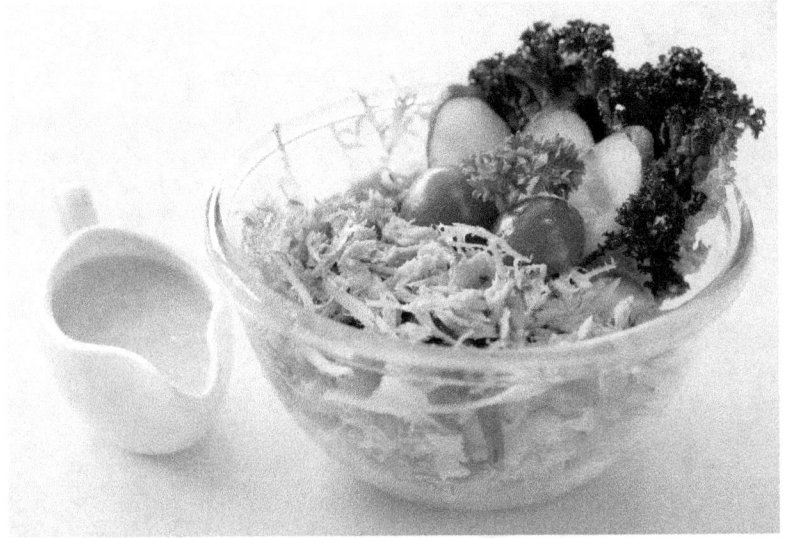

Ingredients:

- 1/3 cup canned coconut milk
- 1 ½ tablespoons Dijon mustard
- 1 teaspoon fresh lemon juice
- Salt and pepper to taste
- 4 (6-ounce) cans tuna in water, drained well
- 1 small seedless cucumber, diced
- ½ cup cherry tomatoes, quartered
- ¼ cup sliced black olives
- ¼ cup diced red onion
- 2 tablespoons roasted red pepper, chopped
- 1 clove minced garlic

Instructions:

1. Combine the coconut milk, mustard and lemon juice in a bowl.
2. Flake the tuna into the bowl and add the remaining ingredients.
3. Toss the salad well to combine then serve over a bed of lettuce.

Roasted Tomato Basil Soup

Servings: 6 to 8

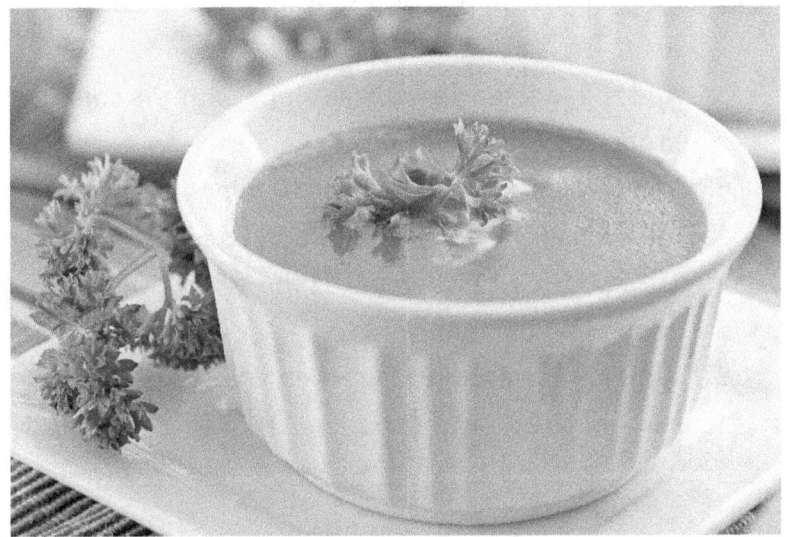

Ingredients:

- 2 lbs. fresh chopped tomatoes
- 1 large yellow onion, sliced thin
- 5 cloves garlic, peeled and sliced
- Olive oil, as needed
- 1 tablespoon coconut oil
- 3 to 4 cups chicken broth
- ½ cup fresh chopped basil
- Salt and pepper to taste
- ½ cup canned coconut milk

Instructions:

1. Preheat the oven to 375°F.
2. Spread the tomatoes, onions and garlic on a rimmed baking sheet and toss with oil.

3. Roast the vegetables for 35 minutes, stirring once, until lightly charred.
4. Heat the coconut oil in a stockpot over medium heat.
5. Add the roasted vegetables along with the chicken broth and bring to a boil.
6. Reduce heat and simmer for 10 minutes then stir in the basil and season with salt and pepper to taste.
7. Turn off the heat then puree the soup with an immersion blender.
8. Whisk in the coconut milk then adjust the seasonings to taste and serve hot.

Chicken, Apple, Pecan Salad

Servings: 6 to 8

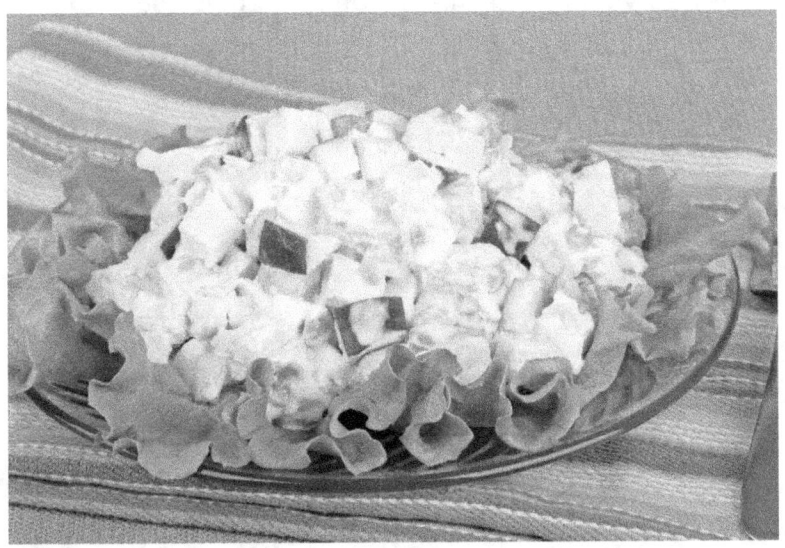

Ingredients:

- 2 lbs. cooked chicken breast, chopped
- 1 large apple, cored and diced
- 2 small stalks celery, sliced thin
- ½ cup chopped pecans
- 1 cup canned coconut milk
- 1 ½ tablespoons Dijon mustard
- 1 teaspoon fresh lemon juice
- Salt and pepper to taste

Instructions:

1. Combine the chicken, apple, celery and pecans in a mixing bowl.
2. In a separate bowl, whisk together the coconut milk, mustard, lemon juice, salt and pepper.

3. Toss the salad with the dressing until evenly coated.
4. Serve the chicken salad on a bed of lettuce.

Cream of Broccoli Soup

Servings: 6 to 8

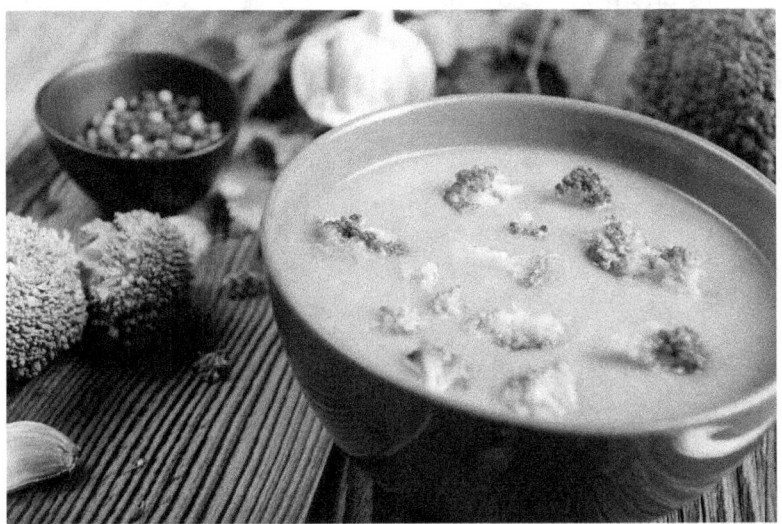

Ingredients:

- 1 tablespoon coconut oil
- 1 small yellow onion, chopped
- 8 cups fresh chopped broccoli
- 1 cup fresh chopped cauliflower
- 1 tablespoon minced garlic
- 3 cups chicken broth
- ½ cup canned coconut milk
- Salt and pepper to taste

Instructions:

1. Heat the oil in a large saucepan over medium-high heat.
2. Add the onion and cook for 5 minutes until translucent.

3. Stir in the broccoli, cauliflower, and garlic.
4. Cook for 5 minutes then stir in the chicken broth and bring to a boil.
5. Reduce heat and simmer for 25 to 30 minutes until the vegetables are tender.
6. Remove from heat and puree the soup using an immersion blender.
7. Whisk in the coconut milk and season the soup with salt and pepper to taste – serve hot.

Strawberry Spinach Salad with Dressing

Servings: 4

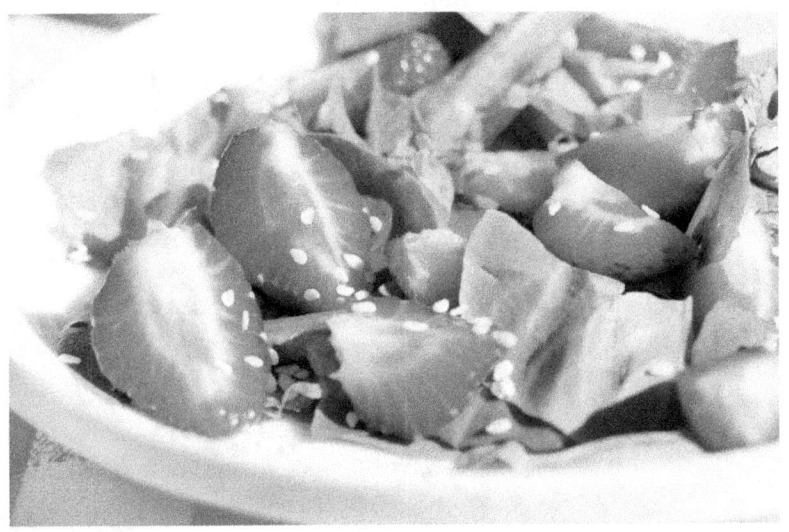

Ingredients:

- 6 cups fresh chopped spinach
- 1 cup sliced mushrooms
- ½ small yellow onion, sliced thin
- 1 ¼ cups fresh diced strawberries, divided
- 2 tablespoons olive oil
- 1 tablespoon balsamic vinegar
- 1 teaspoon honey
- Pinch dry mustard powder
- Salt and pepper to taste
- 2 tablespoons toasted sesame seeds

Instructions:

1. Combine the spinach, mushrooms, and red onion in a large bowl.

2. Add 1 cup diced strawberries and toss to combine.
3. Divide the salad among four plates.
4. Combine the remaining ingredients in a food processor.
5. Blend smooth then drizzle over the salads.
6. Sprinkle the sesame seeds to garnish the salads then serve immediately.

Honey Glazed Carrots

Servings: 6

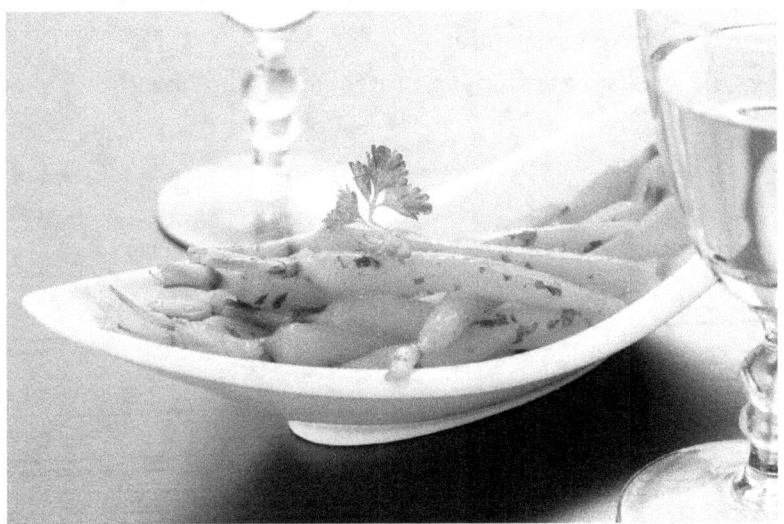

Ingredients:

- 1 ½ cups water
- 1 ½ lbs. carrots, peeled and sliced
- ¼ teaspoon salt
- ¼ cup raw honey
- 2 tablespoons coconut oil
- 1 tablespoon orange zest
- Pinch ground ginger

Instructions:

1. Combine the water, carrots and salt in a medium saucepan.
2. Bring to a boil then reduce heat and simmer on medium for 5 minutes.

3. Drain the carrots then toss in the remaining ingredients.
4. Cook for 2 to 3 minutes, stirring often, until the carrots are tender.
5. Adjust seasonings to taste and serve hot.

Bacon Roasted Brussels Sprouts

Servings: 6 to 8

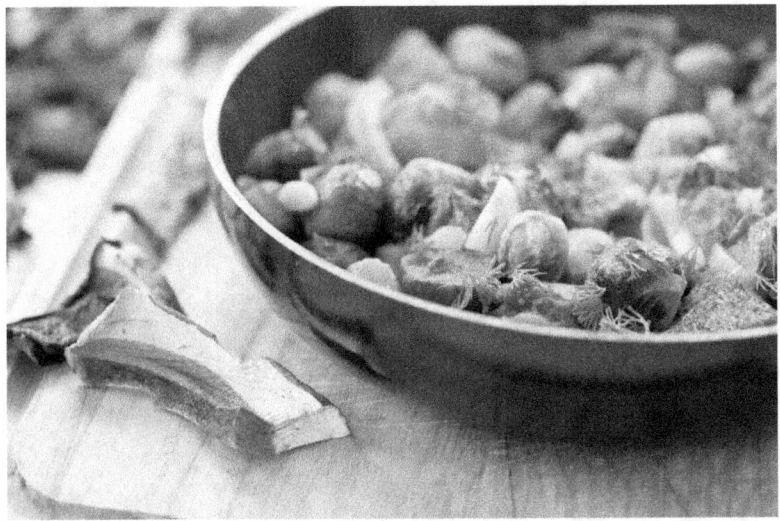

Ingredients:

- 2 lbs. Brussels sprouts, halved
- ¼ cup melted coconut oil
- Salt and pepper to taste
- 6 slices bacon, chopped
- 1 to 2 tablespoons balsamic vinegar

Instructions:

1. Preheat the oven to 400°F.
2. Trim the Brussels sprouts and toss them with the oil then season with salt and pepper to taste.
3. Spread the Brussels sprouts on a rimmed baking sheet and sprinkle with bacon.
4. Roast for 30 minutes, stirring every 10 minutes until tender and browned.

5. Transfer the Brussels sprouts to a serving bowl and drizzle with balsamic vinegar to serve.

Garlic Mashed Cauliflower

Servings: 4

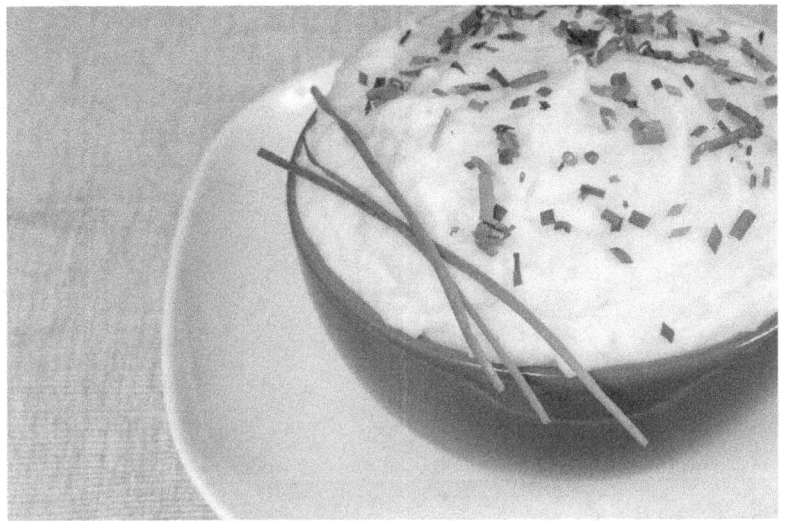

Ingredients:

- 2 to 3 cups water
- 2 medium heads cauliflower, chopped
- 1/3 cup grass-fed butter
- 1 tablespoon minced garlic
- Salt and pepper to taste

Instructions:

1. Bring the water to boil in a saucepan then add the cauliflower, using a steamer insert if you have one.
2. Cover and bring to a boil then steam for 15 to 18 minutes until tender.
3. Transfer the cauliflower to a food processor and pulse to chop.
4. Add the remaining ingredients then blend smooth.

5. Spoon the cauliflower into a bowl and serve hot.

Roasted Rosemary Chicken and Veggies

Servings: 6

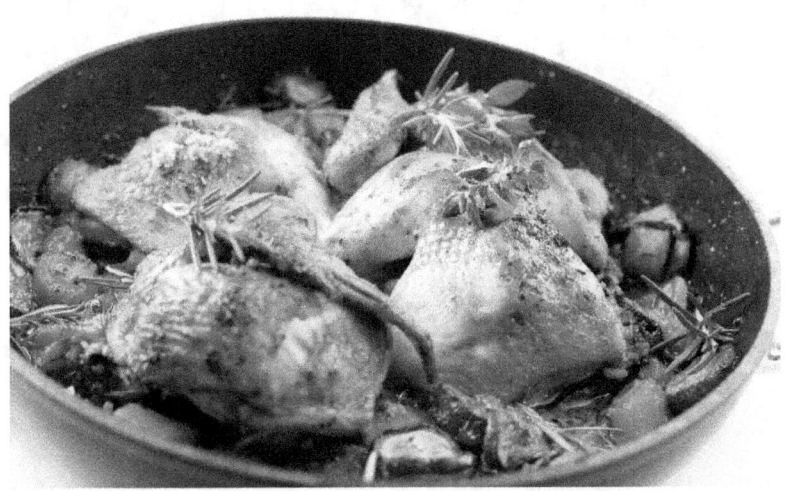

Ingredients:

- 2 tablespoons coconut oil
- 3 lbs. chicken thighs and drumsticks
- Salt and pepper to taste
- 2 large sweet potatoes, peeled and chopped
- 1 large yellow onion, chopped
- 1 small zucchini, sliced thick
- 1 large carrot, peeled and sliced
- 2 tablespoons olive oil
- 1 tablespoon dried rosemary
- ¼ cup chicken broth

Instructions:

1. Preheat the oven to 400°F.

2. Heat the oil in a large skillet over medium-high heat.
3. Season the chicken with salt and pepper to taste then add to the skillet.
4. Cook for 3 to 4 minutes on each side until browned.
5. Combine the veggies in a 9x13-inch glass baking dish and toss with olive oil.
6. Place the chicken on top (skin-side down) and sprinkle with rosemary.
7. Drizzle with chicken broth then roast for 30 minutes.
8. Turn the chicken and stir the veggies then cook for another 25 to 30 minutes until the juices run clear.

Coconut-Crusted Baked Halibut

Servings: 4

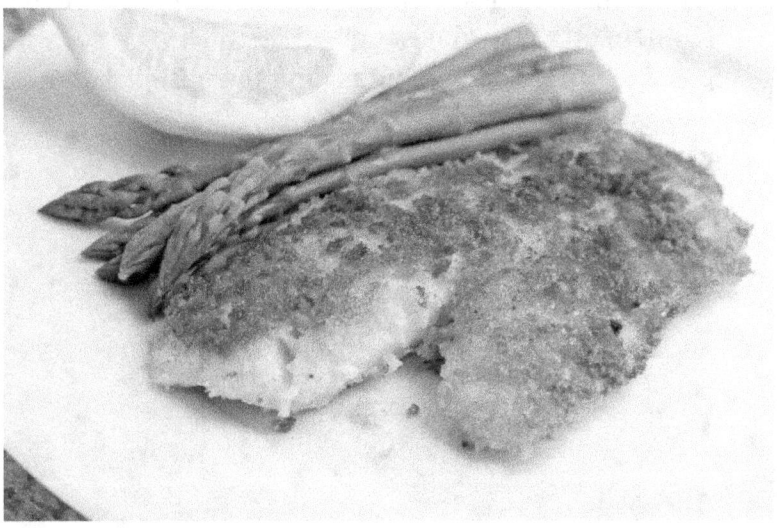

Ingredients:

- 1 large egg, beaten well
- 4 (6-ounce) boneless halibut fillets
- ¼ cup coconut flour
- ½ cup unsweetened shredded coconut
- 1 teaspoon dried parsley
- Salt and pepper to taste
- Lemon wedges

Instructions:

1. Preheat the oven to 350°F and line a baking sheet with parchment.
2. Beat the egg in a shallow dish then dip the fillets in the egg.

3. Combine the coconut flour, coconut, parsley, salt and pepper in a small dish.
4. Dredge the fillets in the coconut mixture then place them on the baking sheet.
5. Bake for 12 to 15 minutes until the flesh flakes easily with a fork.
6. Serve the fillets hot with lemon wedges.

Slow Cooker Beef and Veggie Stew

Servings: 4 to 6

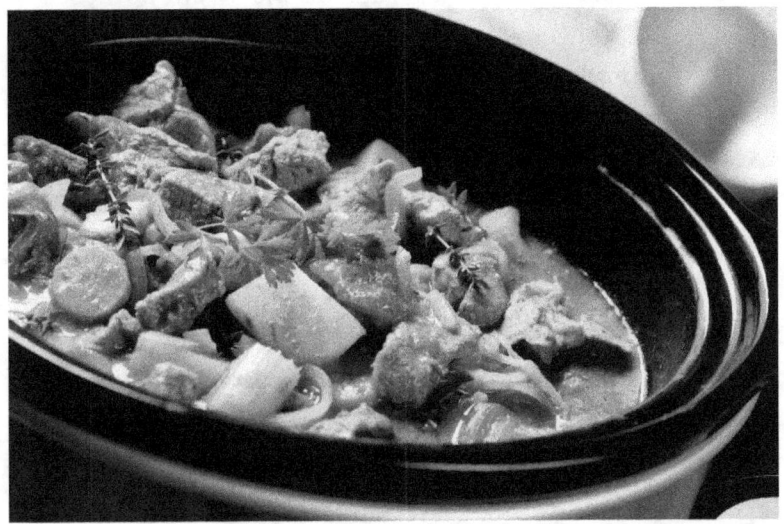

Ingredients:

- 2 tablespoons coconut oil
- 1 large yellow onion, chopped
- 2 large stalks celery, sliced
- 2 large carrots, peeled and sliced
- 2 medium sweet potatoes, peeled and chopped
- 1 ½ lbs. beef stew meat, chopped
- 2 (14.5-ounce) cans diced tomatoes in juice
- 4 cups beef broth
- 1 teaspoon fresh chopped rosemary
- ½ teaspoon fresh chopped thyme
- Salt and pepper to taste

Instructions:

1. Heat the oil in a large Dutch oven over medium-high heat.
2. Add the onion, celery, carrot and sweet potatoes – cook for 5 minutes.
3. Stir in the beef and tomatoes along with the beef broth and seasonings.
4. Cover and simmer the stew for 1 hour, stirring every 15 minutes.
5. Remove the lid and simmer for another 35 to 45 minutes until the vegetables are tender and the beef cooked through.

Fresh Shrimp Ceviche

Servings: 6

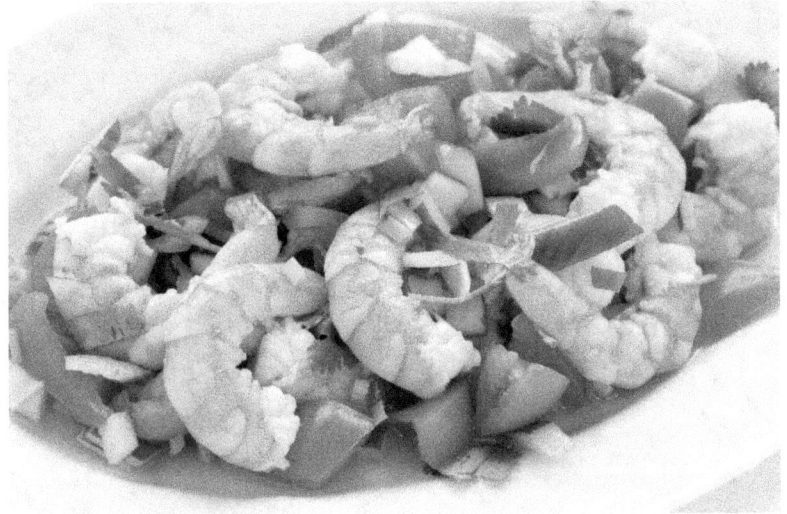

Ingredients:

- 1 ½ cups fresh lime juice
- ¼ cup fresh chopped cilantro
- ¾ lbs. cooked shrimp, peeled and chopped
- 1 small red onion, diced fine
- 2 small seedless cucumbers, diced
- 3 medium tomatoes, cored and diced
- Salt and pepper to taste

Instructions:

1. Whisk together the lime juice and cilantro in a mixing bowl.
2. Toss in the shrimp, red onion, cucumber and tomatoes.
3. Season the ceviche with salt and pepper to taste.

4. Chill until ready to serve.

Garlic Herb Pork Tenderloin

Servings: 4 to 6

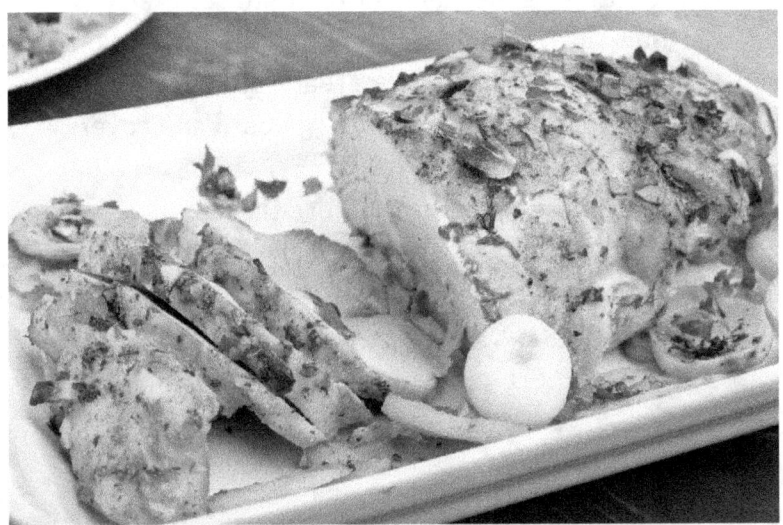

Ingredients:

- 2 (1 to 1 ½ lbs.) boneless pork tenderloins
- Salt and pepper to taste
- 2 tablespoons fresh chopped rosemary
- 2 tablespoons fresh chopped thyme
- 1 tablespoon minced garlic
- 1 tablespoon fresh lemon zest

Instructions:

1. Preheat the oven to 475°F.
2. Season the tenderloins with salt and pepper to taste then place them in a roasting pan.
3. Combine the rosemary, thyme, garlic and lemon zest in a food processor.
4. Blend the mixture into a paste then blend in the oil.

5. Spread the herb and garlic paste over the tenderloins in a thick layer.
6. Roast the tenderloins for ten minutes then flip them and roast for another 8 to 10 minutes until the internal temperature reads 155°F.
7. Remove the pork to a cutting board and cover loosely with foil.
8. Let rest for 10 minutes before slicing.

Coco-Walnut Baked Apples

Servings: 6

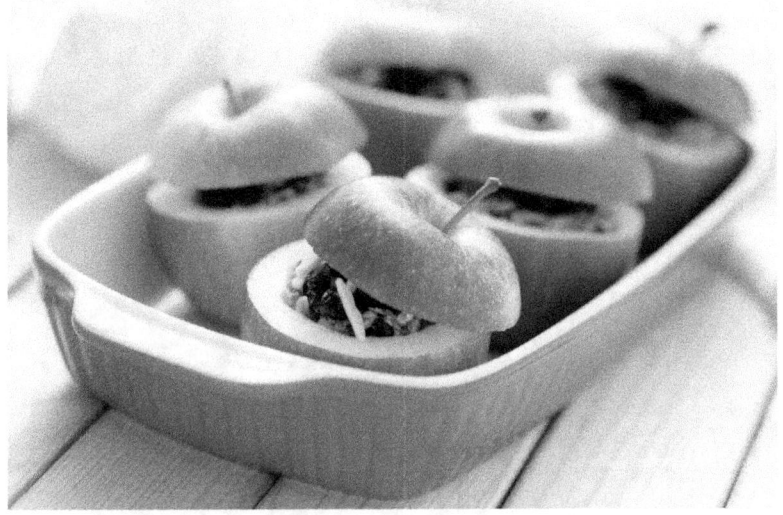

Ingredients:

- 6 ripe apples
- ½ cup seedless raisins
- ¼ cup unsweetened shredded coconut
- 2 tablespoons almond butter
- ½ teaspoon ground cinnamon
- Pinch salt
- 1 cup boiling water

Instructions:

1. Preheat the oven to 375°F.
2. Cut the tops off the apples and scoop out the cores then place the apples upright in a baking dish.
3. Combine the remaining ingredients (except the water) then spoon it into the apples.

4. Pour the water into the dish around the apples.
5. Bake for 35 to 45 minutes until the apples are tender.

Raspberry Fruit Dip

Servings: 6

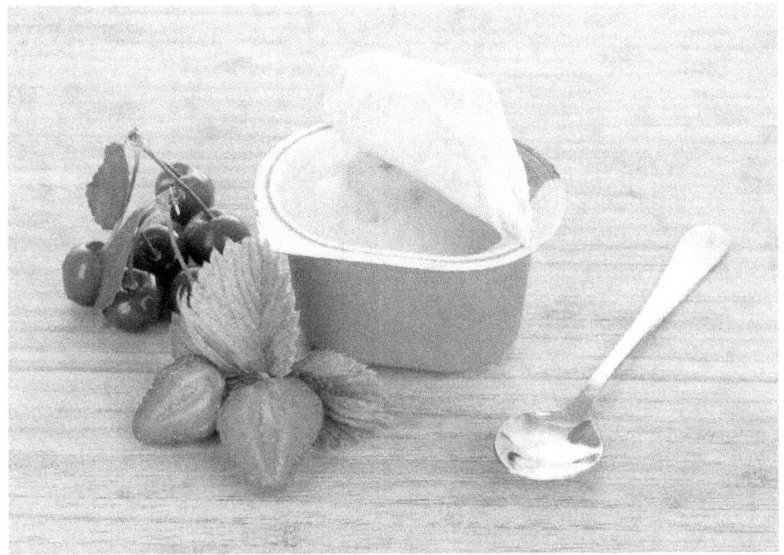

Ingredients:

- 1 ½ cup frozen raspberries, thawed
- 1 ½ cups canned coconut milk
- 3 tablespoons fresh lime juice
- 1 teaspoon fresh lime zest
- 3 tablespoons raw honey

Instructions:

1. Place the raspberries in a food processor and blend smooth.
2. Strain the raspberry puree through a mesh sieve and discard the seeds.
3. Pour the raspberry liquid into a bowl and whisk in the remaining ingredients.

4. Chill the dip then serve with fresh fruit for dipping.

Dairy-Free Banana Ice Cream

Servings: 4

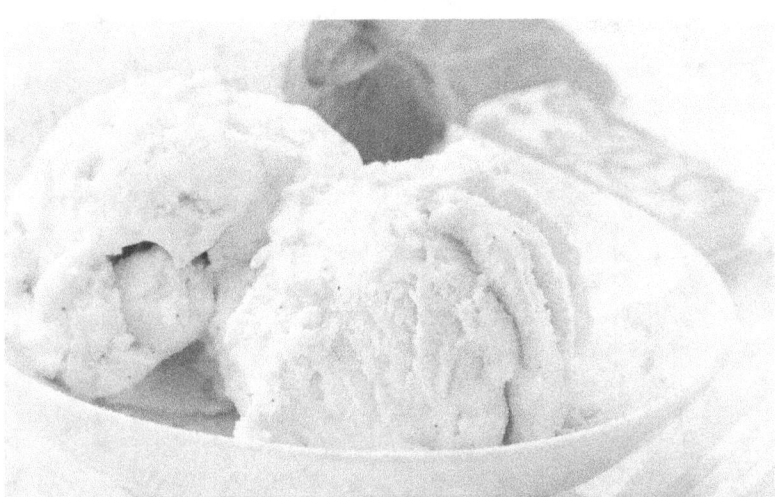

Ingredients:

- 5 large ripe bananas, peeled and sliced

Instructions:

1. Spread the sliced bananas on a parchment-lined baking sheet and freeze overnight.
2. Transfer the slices to a food processor and blend smooth.
3. Spoon the ice cream into bowls and top with fresh fruit or nuts.

Blueberry Almond Crisp

Servings: 6

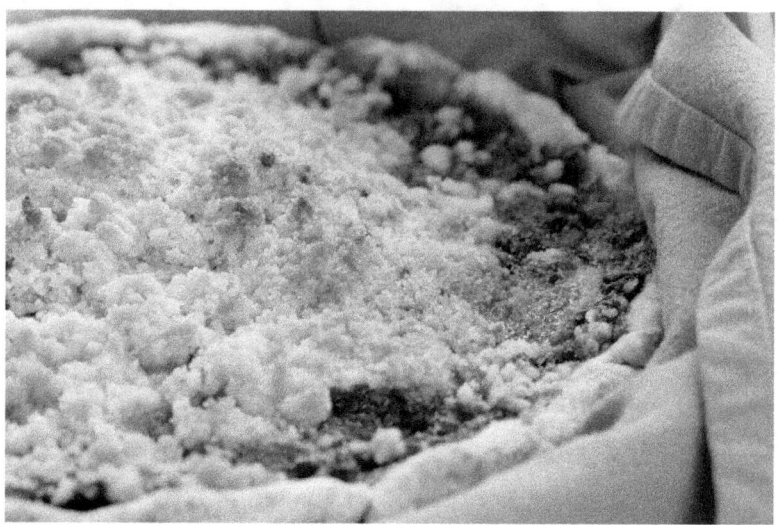

Ingredients:

- 2 lbs. fresh blueberries
- 2 tablespoons raw honey
- 1 teaspoon vanilla extract
- 1 ½ cup raw almonds
- ½ cup unsweetened shredded coconut
- 1 ½ tablespoons maple syrup
- 1 ½ tablespoons coconut milk
- Pinch salt

Instructions:

1. Preheat the oven to 350°F.
2. Combine the blueberries, honey and vanilla in a saucepan over medium-high heat.

3. Bring to a boil then reduce heat and simmer for 10 minutes until thick.
4. Remove from heat and set aside.
5. Combine the almonds and coconut in a food processor.
6. Pulse until finely chopped then blend in the maple syrup, coconut oil and salt.
7. Spoon the berry mixture into a squash glass baking dish and top with the crumble.
8. Bake for 15 minutes or until bubbling and golden brown on top.

No-Bake Coconut Date Balls

Servings: about 2 dozen

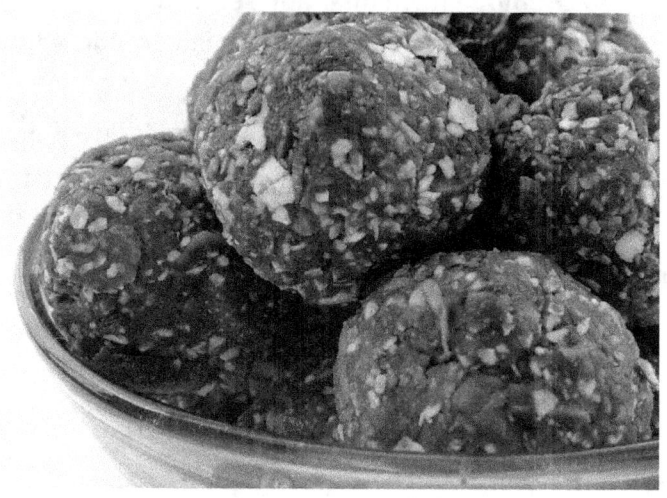

Ingredients:

- 1 cup raw cashews
- 1 cup raw walnuts
- 2 cups seedless raisins
- 6 pitted Medjool dates
- ½ teaspoon vanilla extract
- ¼ teaspoon ground cinnamon

Instructions:

1. Combine the cashews and walnuts in a food processor and pulse to chop.
2. Add the raisins, dates, vanilla and cinnamon.
3. Blend until it forms a stick mixture then roll into 1-inch balls.
4. Roll the balls in the coconut and chill until firm.

Conclusion

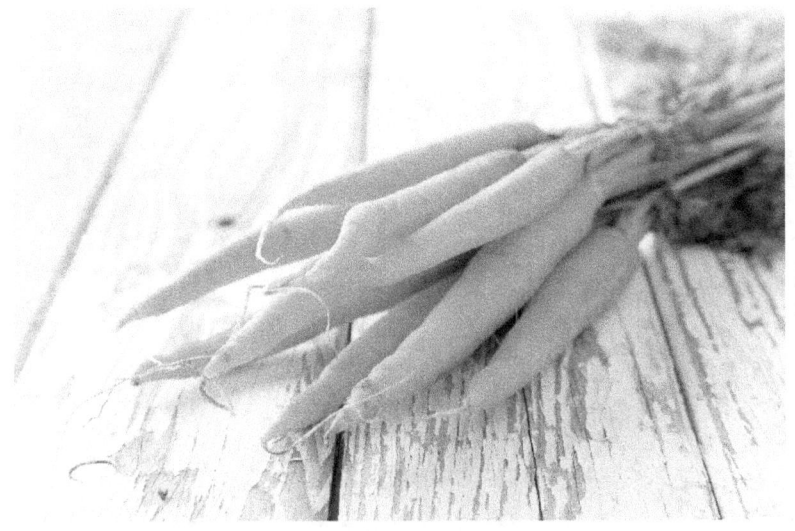

     Just because you are getting older doesn't mean that you have to sit back and allow everything to go south. By taking control of your diet and your eating habits you can do more than just improve your health – you can regain some of your youthful energy and appearance! Switching to the Paleo diet is a great way to increase your consumption of the healthy foods that will help you to fight the signs of aging. You do not have to count calories or restrict your diet in order to achieve your goals – just align your eating habits with the principles of the Paleo diet and, before you know it, you will be looking and feeling younger than ever. If you are ready to transform your life and your body, pick a recipe from this book and get cooking!